The Comprehensive New Mediterranean Diet Cookbook

Easy and Delicious Green Recipes to Enjoy your Meals

GW00644788

Jude Barnes

Table of Contents

Cashew and Bell Pepper Rice

Preparation Time:

5 minutes

Cooking Time:

15minutes

Servings: 2

Ingredients:

- 2 oz. cashew nuts
- ½ yellow bell pepper, deseeded and finely sliced
- 1½ cups cooked basmati rice, cooled
- ½ green bell pepper, deseeded and finely sliced
- ½ small red onion, finely sliced
- For the dressing
- ½ tablespoon brown sugar
- 1 tablespoon light soy sauce
- ¼ lemon, juiced
- 1½ tablespoons mango chutney
- 1 teaspoon curry powder
- ½ tablespoon oil

Directions:

1. Mix together all the ingredients for dressing in a bowl.

2. Toast the cashews until golden brown and transfer to the mixed dressing.

3. Toss in rice, onions and bell peppers and immediately serve.

Nutrition:

- Calories 433
- Total Fat 17.1 g
- Saturated Fat 3.2 g
- Cholesterol 0 mg
- Total Carbs 70.6 g
- Dietary Fiber 2.5 g
- Sugar 14.1 g
- Protein 10.3 g

Roasted Vegetable Tabbouleh

Preparation Time:

5 minutes

Cooking Time:

35 minutes

Servings: 2

Ingredients:

- 1 (8-ounce) can garbanzo beans, rinsed and drained
- ¼ cup fresh parsley, chopped
- 2 small carrots, chopped
- 1/3 cup bulgur, boiled and drained
- ½ small red onion, chopped
- 1½ tablespoons lemon juice
- ¼ teaspoon black pepper
- ¼ teaspoon lemon peel, finely shredded
- 1 tablespoon water
- ½ medium tomatoes, chopped
- 1 tablespoon olive oil
- 1/8 teaspoon salt
- 1 teaspoon fresh thyme, snipped

Directions:

1. Preheat the oven to 390 degrees F and lightly grease a baking dish.
2. Organize carrots and onions in a baking dish and drizzle with olive oil.
3. Bake for about 25 minutes and dish out in a bowl.
4. Add lemon peel, pepper, salt, bulgur, parsley, lemon juice and garbanzo to the baked veggies bowl and immediately serve.

Nutrition:

- Calories 370
- Total Fat 10.6 g
- Saturated Fat 1.5 g
- Cholesterol 0 mg
- Total Carbs 58.7 g
- Dietary Fiber 15.9 g
- Sugar 9.6 g
- Protein 14.1 g

Moroccan Couscous

Preparation Time:

5 minutes

Cooking Time:

20 minutes

Servings: 16

Ingredients:

- 2/3 cup dried apricots, chopped
- 2 oranges, juiced
- 2/3 cup golden raisins
- 1 teaspoon ground ginger
- 2 oranges, zested
- ½ teaspoon ground cinnamon
- 3 cups vegetable stock
- 2/3 cup dates, chopped
- 1 teaspoon ground cumin
- 4 cups whole-wheat couscous
- 1 cup slivered almonds, toasted
- ½ teaspoon coriander
- 2 tablespoons butter
- Salt, to taste
- 1 teaspoon turmeric
- ½ cup mint, chopped

Directions:

1. Boil stock in a saucepan and add orange juice, zest, dates, apricots, raisins, couscous and spices.

2. Remove the pan from heat and allow the couscous to absorb the liquid for about 15 minutes.

3. Stir in the butter, mint and almonds and sprinkle with salt to serve.

Nutrition:

- Calories 264
- Total Fat 5 g
- Saturated Fat 1 g
- Cholesterol 4 mg
- Total Carbs 48 g
- Dietary Fiber 4 g
- Sugar 7.5 g
- Protein 8 g

Parmesan Roasted Broccoli

Preparation Time:

5 minutes

Cooking Time:

35 minutes

Servings: 8

Ingredients:

- 1 cup Parmesan cheese, grated
- 2 pounds broccoli florets, cut into bite-sized pieces
- 4 tablespoons olive oil
- 2 lemons, zested
- ¼ teaspoon sea salt
- Salt, to taste
- ¼ teaspoon red pepper flakes
- 4 tablespoons balsamic vinegar

Directions:

1. Preheat the oven to 395 degrees F and lightly grease a baking sheet.
2. Season the broccoli florets with salt and place on the baking sheet.
3. Bake for about 15 minutes and top with parmesan cheese.
4. Bake these florets again for about 10 minutes and dish out in a bowl.

5. Season with lemon zest, salt, red pepper flakes and balsamic vinegar to serve.

Nutrition:

- Calories 146
- Total Fat 10.4 g
- Saturated Fat 3 g
- Cholesterol 10 mg
- Total Carbs 8.5 g
- Dietary Fiber 3 g
- Sugar 2.4 g
- Protein 7.7 g

Spinach Beans

Preparation Time:

10 minutes

Cooking Time:

30 minutes

Servings: 4

Ingredients:

- 2 cans (14½ ounces) diced tomatoes, undrained
- 2 cans (15 ounces) cannellini beans, rinsed and drained
- 4 garlic cloves, minced
- ½ teaspoon black pepper
- 28 ounces bacon, chopped
- 2 small onions, chopped
- ½ teaspoon salt
- 12 ounces fresh baby spinach
- 2 tablespoons olive oil
- 4 tablespoons Worcestershire sauce
- ¼ teaspoon red pepper flakes, crushed

Directions:

1. Heat oil in a skillet on medium heat and add bacon.
2. Sauté until brown and stir in the garlic and onions.

3. Sauté for about 5 minutes and add Worcestershire sauce, seasonings and tomatoes.

4. Reduce the heat and cook for about 10 minutes.

5. Toss in the beans and spinach and cook for about 5 minutes.

6. Stir well and serve immediately.

Nutrition:

- Calories 475
- Total Fat 8.5 g
- Saturated Fat 1.2 g
- Cholesterol 0 mg
- Total Carbs 77.8 g
- Dietary Fiber 31.1 g
- Sugar 10.1 g
- Protein 28.2 g

Roasted Carrots Recipe

Preparation Time:

5 min

Cooking Time:

30 min

Servings: 6

Ingredients:

- ½ tablespoon of a lime juice
- ½ teaspoon of ground turmeric
- Kosher Salt
- 1 finely minced garlic clove
- Black pepper
- Extra virgin olive oil
- 2 lb. peeled carrots
- Parsley

Directions:

1. Preheat the oven at 400 degrees F and get a large mixing bowl. Pour the sliced carrots in it and spray it with extra virgin olive oil.
2. Stir to ensure that the oil circulates to the carrots, then spice it with salt and pepper.
3. Arrange the carrots into a baking sheet and cook for about 20 min.

4. Turn them at about half time to ensure that the color remains balanced on both sides.

5. Then take it out of the oven and serve. Here is the time to season with your turmeric and garnish with fresh parsley.

Nutrition:

- 67.5 kcal
- 0.7g of fat
- 4.6g of fiber
- 0.7mg of iron
- 51.4mg of calcium
- 13.2g of carbs
- 1.98g of protein.

Homemade Pita Chips

Preparation Time:

5 minutes

Cooking Time:

10 min

Servings: 6

Ingredients:

- 2 pita breads that have pockets
- Kosher salt
- Extra virgin olive oil
- Use any seasoning.

Directions:

1. Preheat the oven at 430 degrees F and get a large baking sheet near. Get a large cutting board and place each pita on it.
2. Use kitchen shears to cut them into halves, you can equally use a knife.
3. I advise you should not use the thick single layered pitas so that you can easily follow this step.
4. If that's what you are using, however, do not bother to cut it into halves.
5. Stroke all sides of the pita with the extra virgin olive oil and add your salt to it.

6. Brush it with your seasoning too.

7. Take each pita and cut into 8 triangles and place them in the baking sheet.

8. Bake for about 7 min and turn it over once in a while to ensure that the colors on the two sides are balanced.

Nutrition:

- 14.4 kcal
- 0.3g of fat
- 27mg of sodium
- 5mg of calcium
- 0.3mg of Iron
- 2.8g of carbs
- 0.5g of protein.

Pressure Pot Hummus

Preparation Time:

10 minutes

Cooking Time:

1 hour

Servings: 6-8

Ingredients:

- 1 cup dried chickpeas
- 1 head of garlic, crushed
- 2 bay leaves
- 1 onion, cut in half
- 1 1/2 teaspoon fine salt
- 4 cups of cold water
- 1 teaspoon ground cumin
- 6 garlic cloves, crushed
- 1 cup tahini
- 1/4 cup lemon juice

Directions:

1. Rinse chickpeas thoroughly under cold water.
2. Add chickpeas, bay leaves, garlic head, and onion half into the Pressure Pot. Add salt.

3. Pour in water, and mix. Place knob to a venting position, close the lid, and turn the knob to sealing position.

4. Cook and then natural release for 20 minutes. Open the lid carefully.

5. Soak 6 cloves of garlic in freshly squeezed lemon juice in a blender for 20-30 minutes before blending. Discard the onions and bay leaves.

6. Drain the chickpeas and garlic cloves well and then set aside chickpeas and liquid. Blend the garlic and lemon juice in a blender.

7. Add chickpeas, cooked garlic clove, ground cumin, and 3/4 cup chickpea liquid to the garlic lemon juice in the blender.

8. Blend the chickpeas at the lowest speed, and then increase slowly to high speed. Blend until smooth

9. Season with salt to taste.

Nutrition:

- Calories: 293
- Protein: 11 g
- Total Fat: 18 g
- Carbohydrates: 27 g

Pressure Pot Tomato Sauce

Preparation Time:

10 minutes

Cooking Time:

50 minutes

Servings: 3 cups

Ingredients:

- 4 medium ripe tomatoes, chopped
- 1 small onion, peeled, trimmed at the root, and cut in half
- 6 tablespoons butter
- 4 sprigs basil
- 1 teaspoon sea salt

Directions:

1. Merge all of the ingredients and place the valve to sealing, and then push manual high pressure to adjust the time to 8 minutes.
2. Push "Keep Warm/Cancel" to turn off warming mode. Quick-release the pressure. When finished, remove the lid.
3. Puree the sauce in a blender until you reach your desired consistency. Leave the onion in while blending, or remove.

Nutrition:

- Calories: 121
- Protein: 1 g
- Total Fat: 12 g
- Carbohydrates: 4 g

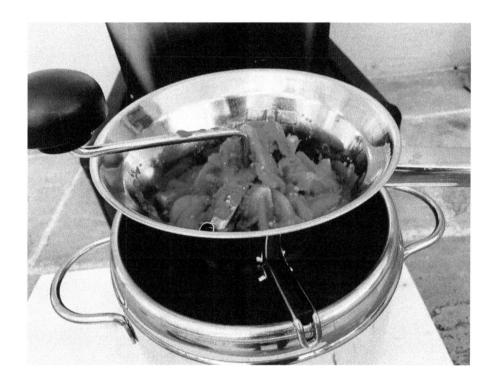

Pressure Pot Homemade Spaghetti Sauce

Preparation Time:

10 minutes

Cooking Time:

25 minutes

Servings: 6

Ingredients:

- 1 pound ground Italian sausage
- 1 yellow onion, diced
- 1 cup beef broth
- 28 ounce can crushed tomatoes
- 14 1/2 ounce can diced tomatoes
- 2 tablespoons tomato paste
- 1 bay leaf
- 2 teaspoons dried basil
- 1 teaspoon garlic powder
- 1/2 teaspoon dried oregano
- 1 teaspoon brown sugar
- Salt and pepper

Directions:

1. Set up your Pressure Pot and then add the sausage when heated.
2. Use a wooden spoon to move sausage around and brown on all sides.
3. Add in onions and let them soften for 3 minutes.
4. Deglaze the pot with beef broth, and then add all of the tomatoes, tomato paste, bay leaf, basil, garlic powder, oregano, and brown sugar.
5. Cover the pot and secure the lid. Make sure the valve setting is sealing.
6. Set manual to high pressure and cook for 10 minutes.
7. Remove the lid carefully and stir the sauce.
8. Discard bay leaf and add salt and pepper to taste.
9. The sauce is now ready.

Nutrition:

- Calories: 145
- Protein: 7 g
- Total Fat: 9 g
- Carbohydrates: 8 g

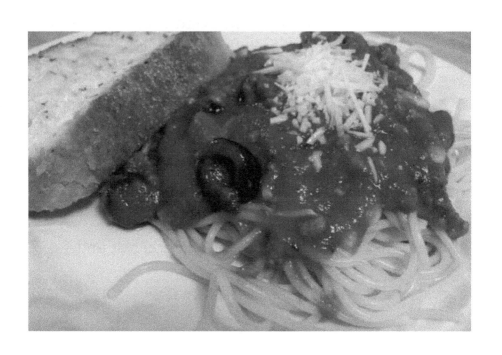

Pressure Pot Sicilian Meat Sauce

Preparation Time:

10 minutes

Cooking Time:

70 minutes

Servings: 6

Ingredients:

- 3 tablespoons olive oil
- 2 pounds boneless pork ribs, trimmed
- 1 onion, chopped
- 5 garlic cloves, minced
- 28-ounce cans diced tomatoes
- 1 can Italian tomato paste
- 3 bay leaves
- 2 tablespoons fresh parsley, chopped
- 2 tablespoons capers, chopped
- 1/2 teaspoon dried basil
- 1/2 teaspoon crushed dried rosemary
- 1/2 teaspoon dried thyme
- 1/2 teaspoon crushed red pepper flakes
- 1/2 teaspoon salt
- 1/2 teaspoon sugar
- 1 cup beef broth
- 1/2 cup dry red wine

Directions:

1. Select the sauté option on Pressure Pot and add 2 tablespoons of olive oil. Then remove and set aside.
2. Add remaining oil, sauté onion for 2 minutes, then add garlic and cook for another minute.
3. Add the remaining ingredients and then transfer the meat back to the Pressure Pot.
4. Pour in the broth and red wine, and bring to a boil. Lock the lid and adjust to manual high pressure for 35 minutes.
5. Once cooking is processed, release gently for 10 minutes and then quickly release the rest of the pressure.
6. Remove meat from the pressure cooker, shred, discard bone, and return the meat to the sauce.
7. Serve over your favorite pasta.

Nutrition:

- Calories: 214
- Protein: 16 g
- Total Fat: 11 g
- Carbohydrates: 13 g

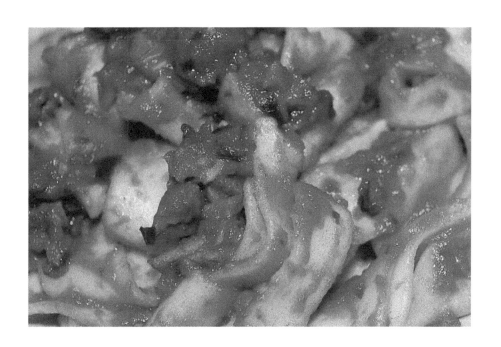

Pressure Pot Cranberry Sauce

Preparation Time:

10 minutes

Cooking Time:

50 minutes

Servings: 3

Ingredients:

- 12-ounce packages fresh cranberries
- 1/2 cup brown sugar
- 1/2 cup freshly squeezed orange juice
- 2 strips orange zest
- 1 cinnamon stick
- 1/4 teaspoon ground cloves
- 1/2 teaspoon vanilla extract

Directions:

1. Place the cranberries, sugar, orange juice, orange zest, cinnamon, and cloves into your Pressure Pot.
2. Stir well.
3. Select manual high pressure and set a timer for 4 minutes.
4. Allow the natural release of pressure, 20 minutes.
5. Remove the orange zest and cinnamon using a wooden spoon.

6. Mash cranberry mixture until you reach the desired consistency.

7. Stir in vanilla and let it cool completely.

Nutrition:

- Calories: 86
- Protein: 0.1 g
- Total Fat: 0.1 g
- Carbohydrates: 22 g

Pressure Pot Applesauce

Preparation Time:

10 minutes

Cooking Time:

20 minutes

Servings: 4

Ingredients:

- 3 pounds apples
- Juice from 1 lemon
- 1/2 cup of water
- 1 cinnamon stick

Directions:

1. Peel the apples, core, and cut into 8 slices
2. Place the apples at the bottom of the Pressure Pot; add lemon juice, water, and cinnamon.
3. Attach the lid and put it in the sealing position. Set on manual high pressure for 6 minutes.
4. Once processed, release naturally for 6 minutes. Quick-release the remainder of pressure. Remove lid carefully, let it cool, and remove the cinnamon stick.
5. Mash with a potato masher. It is now ready to serve.

Nutrition:

- Calories: 90
- Protein: 0.4 g
- Total Fat: 0.2 g
- Carbohydrates: 24.1 g

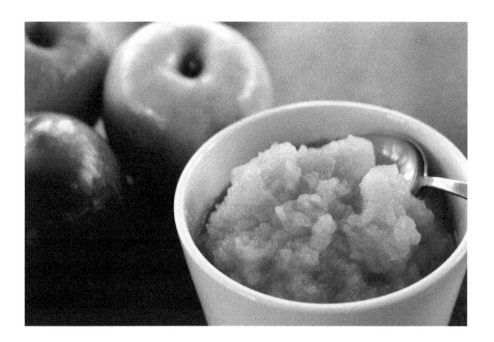

Pressure Pot Spicy Curry Hummus

Preparation Time:

10 minutes

Cooking Time:

30 minutes

Servings: 12

Ingredients:

- 1 1/2 cups garbanzo beans, dry
- 4 cups of water
- 1/3 cup tahini
- 1/4 cup extra-virgin olive oil
- 2 cloves garlic, peeled
- 1 tablespoon curry powder
- 1 teaspoon turmeric
- 1/4 teaspoon cayenne
- 1 lemon, juiced
- Salt and pepper

Directions:

1. Oak garbanzo beans overnight.
2. Attach garbanzo beans along with 4 cups of water to your Pressure Pot.
3. Set the Pressure Pot to high pressure for 25 minutes.
4. When cooking complete, allow pressure to release naturally.

5. Then quick release to relieve any remaining pressure.
6. Let the garbanzo beans cool a bit.
7. Merge the garbanzo beans, tahini, olive oil, garlic, curry, turmeric, cayenne, lemon juice, salt, and pepper.
8. Blend until creamy.
9. Hummus ready for serving

Nutrition:

- Calories: 372
- Protein: 16.7
- Total Fat: 12.9
- Carbohydrates: 50.9

Pressure Pot Tahini Cashew Curry Recipe

Preparation Time:

10 minutes

Cooking Time:

15 minutes

Servings: 2

Ingredients:

- 2 cups unsweetened cashew milk
- 2 tablespoons tahini paste
- 2 teaspoons curry paste
- 2 teaspoons fresh minced ginger
- ½ teaspoon sea salt
- 1 tablespoon turmeric
- 1 tablespoon tapioca starch
- 1 cup cauliflower florets
- ½ cup onion, chopped
- ½ red bell pepper, chopped

Directions:

1. Whisk the cashew milk, tahini paste, curry paste, ginger, sea salt, turmeric together into the Pressure Pot.
2. Set on sauté mode and bring it to a boil.

3. Stir in cauliflower, onions, and pepper into the Pressure Pot.

4. Set it to sealing and cook on manual high pressure for 1 minute.

5. Let pressure release naturally.

6. Serve over rice or with pita bread.

Nutrition:

- Calories: 232
- Protein: 5 g
- Total Fat: 15 g
- Carbohydrates: 20 g

Pressure Pot Mediterranean Pizza Dip

Preparation Time:

10 minutes

Cooking Time:

35 minutes

Servings: 8

Ingredients:

- 8-ounce package of cream cheese
- 8 ounces Monterey Jack cheese, shredded
- 1 cup cherry tomatoes, chopped
- ¾ cup boneless ham steak, chopped
- ½ sliced black olives
- ½ cup marinated artichoke hearts, chopped
- 3 ounces crumbled feta cheese
- 3 cloves garlic, pressed
- ½ tablespoon chopped fresh basil
- 1 teaspoon Italian seasoning

Directions:

1. Combine the cream cheese, Monterey Jack, cherry tomatoes, ham steak, olives, artichoke hearts, feta cheese, garlic, basil, and Italian seasoning in a bowl and mix well.

2. Pour into a rounding glass baking dish and cover with aluminum foil. Make sure the dish will fit inside the Pressure Pot.
3. Whisk 1 cup of water.
4. Set the metal trivet inside and place the baking dish on top.
5. Cover and cook.
6. Release the pressure using quick release.
7. Carefully unlock and remove the lid.
8. Stir and serve.

Nutrition:

- Calories: 285
- Protein: 14.1 g
- Total Fat: 23.9 g
- Carbohydrates: 4.3 g

Pressure Pot Marinara Sauce with Fresh Tomatoes

Preparation Time:

10 minutes

Cooking Time:

35 minutes

Servings: 16 ounces jars

Ingredients:

- 1 pound tomatoes, diced
- 1 large onion, diced
- 8 garlic cloves, minced
- 1 tablespoon dried basil
- 1 tablespoon dried oregano
- 1 diced carrot
- 2 tablespoons fresh basil, chopped
- 2 tablespoons fresh parsley, chopped
- 4 ounces vegetable broth
- 2 tablespoon olive oil
- Salt to taste

Directions:

1. Heat the pot and add the olive oil to heat.
2. Attach the garlic, and cook, then add the dried herbs and onions.

3. Sauté for a couple of minutes until you smell the garlicups

4. Throw in the tomatoes, carrots, fresh herbs, and broth.

5. Close the lid and seal the vent. Pressure cook on high for 15 minutes.

6. Blend all the ingredients and process until you reach your desired consistency.

7. It is now ready to serve.

Nutrition:

- Calories: 65
- Protein: 1.8 g
- Total Fat: 1.9 g
- Carbohydrates: 10 g

Pressure Pot Chickpeas Curry

Preparation Time:

10 minutes

Cooking Time:

11 hours

Servings: 15

Ingredients:

- 1 cup dried chickpeas
- 1 tablespoon olive oil
- 1 tablespoon cumin seeds
- 1 tablespoon crushed ginger
- 4 cloves garlic, crushed
- 1 chopped onion
- 2 green chilies, deseeded
- 2 aroma tomatoes, finely chopped
- 1 teaspoon salt
- 1 tablespoon coriander powder
- 1 tablespoon garam masala
- 1 teaspoon cumin powder
- 1/4 teaspoon cayenne
- 1 teaspoon red chili powder
- 1/2 teaspoon fennel powder
- 2 cups water

Directions:

1. First, rinse and soak the chickpeas overnight in 4 cups of water. Strain them and rinse thoroughly.

2. Turn the Pressure Pot to sauté setting and add cumin seeds after 30 seconds.

3. When the cumin begins to sputter, add onions, garlic, and ginger, green chilies, tomato, and sauté for a minute.

4. Add the spices, chickpeas, and water. Close the lid, set to sealing, and pressure cook for 35 minutes at bean setting.

5. When processed, naturally release the pressure for 10 minutes, and then quickly release the remainder of the pressure.

6. Open the lid and remove contents. Smash few beans to make the curry creamier. May garnish with cumin powder and squeeze some fresh lemon juice.

7. It is now ready to serve.

Nutrition:

- Calories: 205
- Protein: 9 g
- Total Fat: 6 g
- Carbohydrates: 31 g

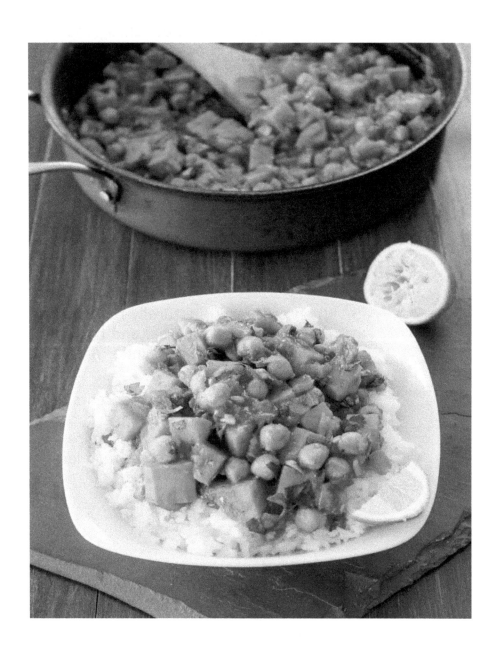

Pressure Pot Sweet Chili Sauce

Preparation Time:

10 minutes

Cooking Time:

35 minutes

Servings: 16

Ingredients:

- 2 fresh long chili peppers, halved
- 2 garlic cloves, peeled
- 1-inch peeled ginger
- 1/2 cup water
- 1/2 cup apple cider vinegar
- 1/2 cup mild honey
- Salt to taste

Directions:

1. Place the chili peppers, garlic, and ginger in a food processor and process until finely chopped.
2. Press the sauté button on the Pressure
3. Pot and let sit until heated, add the chili mixture, water, vinegar, and honey, and mix thoroughly.
4. Cook and occasionally stir until the sauce thickness is to your liking for 15-20 minutes.

5. Add salt to taste.

6. Transfer the sauce to a jar.

Nutrition:

- Calories: 37
- Protein: 0.2 g
- Total Fat: 0
- Carbohydrates: 9.6 g

Pressure Pot Roasted Red Pepper Sauce

Preparation Time:

10 minutes

Cooking Time:

45 minutes

Servings: 4

Ingredients:

- 1 teaspoon coconut oil
- 1 onion
- 3 cloves garlic
- 1/2 teaspoon coriander
- 1/2 teaspoon cumin
- 1/2 teaspoon black pepper
- 1/8 teaspoon Ceylon cinnamon
- 1 can diced tomatoes
- 3 roasted red bell peppers, chopped
- 2 teaspoons of apple cider vinegar
- 1 teaspoon chili garlic paste
- 1/2 teaspoon paprika powder
- 1/4 teaspoons ancho chili powder
- 1 teaspoon salt

Directions:

1. Heat the pot to sauté mode and melt the coconut oil.
2. Fry the onions for 7 minutes until translucent, then add garlic and fry for another minute.
3. Merge some more coconut oil to one corner of the pot and sprinkle the coriander, cumin, black pepper, and Ceylon cinnamon into the same corner.
4. Fry for 30 seconds and stir well.
5. Add diced tomatoes, bell peppers, vinegar, chili garlic paste, paprika, salt, and chili.
6. Close the lid, turn to sealing, and set the Pressure Pot into pressure cooking mode for 10 minutes.
7. Quick-release the pressure and transfer the sauce into a blender. Blend until smooth.

Nutrition:

- Calories: 336
- Protein: 1.9 g
- Total Fat: 31 g
- Carbohydrates: 12 g

Pressure Pot Ace Blender Beef Marinade

Preparation Time:

10 minutes

Cooking Time:

9 minutes

Servings: 2.5 cups

Ingredients:

- 3/4 cup tomato juice
- 1 1/2 cups balsamic vinegar
- 2 tablespoon Worcestershire sauce
- 2 tablespoons olive oil
- 1 1/2 teaspoon ground black pepper
- 1 1/2 kosher salt
- 1/2 teaspoon dried thyme
- 3 cloves of garlic
- 1/2 yellow onion

Directions:

1. Add all of the ingredients to an Pressure Pot Ace Blender. Secure the lid and select pulse.
2. Blend until smooth.

Nutrition:

- Calories: 9.9
- Protein: 0 g
- Total Fat: 0 g
- Carbohydrates: 2 g

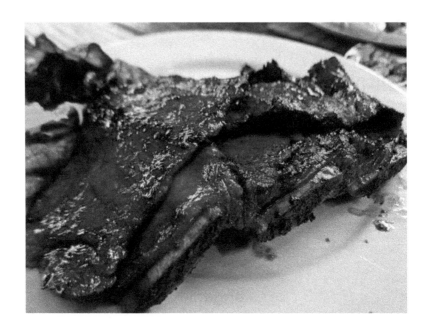

Ace Blender Tuscan White Bean Dip

Preparation Time:

10 minutes

Cooking Time:

6 minutes

Servings: 3 cups

Ingredients:

- 3 teaspoons fresh basil
- 30 ounces cannellini beans
- 2 cloves garlic
- 1/4 yellow onion, diced
- 1/4 cup vegetable stock
- 1 teaspoon Italian seasoning
- 1/2 teaspoon black pepper
- 1/2 teaspoon salt
- 1/4 cup extra-virgin olive oil
- 1/3 cup grated Parmesan cheese

Directions:

1. Place all ingredients in an Pressure Pot Ace Blender. Pulse until smooth.
2. Pour into a bowl and it is ready to serve.

Nutrition:

- Calories: 34.5
- Protein: 2.4 g
- Total Fat: 0.2 g
- Carbohydrates: 6.3 g

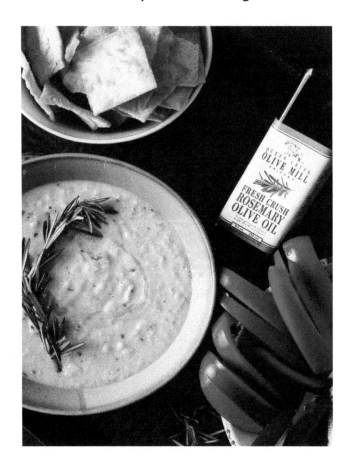

Melon Salad

Preparation Time:

10 minutes

Cooking Time:

20 minutes

Servings: 6

Ingredients:

- 1/4 teaspoon sea salt
- 1/4 teaspoon black pepper
- 1 tablespoon balsamic vinegar
- 1 cantaloupe, quartered and seeded
- 12 watermelon, small and seedless
- 2 cups mozzarella balls, fresh
- 1/3 cup basil, fresh and torn
- 2 tablespoons olive oil

Directions:

1. Get out a melon baller and scoop out balls of cantaloupe, and then put them in a colander over a serving bowl.

2. Use your melon baller to cut the watermelon as well, and then put them in with your cantaloupe.

3. Allow your fruit to drain for ten minutes, and then refrigerate the juice for another recipe.

4. It can even be added to smoothies.

5. Wipe the bowl dry, and then place your fruit in it.

6. Add in your basil, oil, vinegar, mozzarella, and tomatoes before seasoning with salt and pepper.

7. Gently mix and serve immediately or chilled.

Nutrition:

- Calories: 218
- Protein: 10 g
- Fat: 13 g
- Carbs: 17 g

Orange Celery Salad

Preparation Time:

5 minutes

Cooking Time:

15 minutes

Servings: 6

Ingredients:

- 1 tablespoon lemon juice, fresh
- 1/4 teaspoon sea salt, fine
- 1/4 teaspoon black pepper
- 1 tablespoon olive brine
- 1 tablespoon olive oil
- 1/4 cup red onion, sliced
- 1/2 cup green olives
- 2 oranges, peeled and sliced
- 3 celery stalks, sliced diagonally in 1/2 inch slices

Directions:

1. Put your oranges, olives, onion, and celery in a shallow bowl.
2. In a different bowl whisk your oil, olive brine, and lemon juice, pour this over your salad.
3. Season with salt and pepper before serving.

Nutrition:

- Calories: 65
- Protein: 2 g
- Fat: 0 g
- Carbs: 9 g

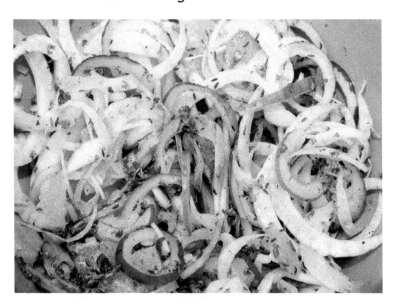

Roasted Broccoli Salad

Preparation Time:

30 minutes

Cooking Time:

30 minutes

Servings: 4

Ingredients:

- 1 pound broccoli, cut into florets, and stem sliced
- 3 tablespoons olive oil, divided
- 1 pint cherry tomatoes
- 1 1/2 teaspoons honey, raw and divided
- 3 cups cubed bread, whole grain
- 1 tablespoon balsamic vinegar
- 1/2 teaspoon black pepper
- 1/4 teaspoon sea salt, fine
- Grated Parmesan for serving

Directions:

1. Preheat your oven.
2. Drizzle your broccoli with a tablespoon of oil, and toss to coat.
3. Remove the baking sheet from the oven, and spoon the broccoli on it.

4. Leave oil at the bottom of the bowl, and add in your tomatoes, toss to coat, and then toss your tomatoes with a tablespoon of honey.

5. Pour them on the same baking sheet as your broccoli.

6. Roast for fifteen minutes, and stir halfway through your cooking Time.

7. Add in your bread, and then roast for three more minutes.

8. Whisk two tablespoons of oil, vinegar, and remaining honey.

9. Season with salt and pepper. Pour this over your broccoli mix to serve.

Nutrition:

- Calories: 226
- Protein: 7 g
- Fat: 12 g
- Carbohydrates: 26 g

Leeks Cream

Preparation Time:

5 minutes

Cooking Time:

30 minutes

Servings: 4

Ingredients:

- 4 sliced leeks
- 4 cups vegetable stock
- 1 tablespoon olive oil
- 2 chopped shallots
- 1 tablespoon chopped rosemary
- Pinch of salt
- Black pepper
- 1 cup heavy cream
- 1 tablespoon chopped chives

Directions:

1. Heat up a pot with the oil over medium-high heat; add the shallots and the leeks and sauté for 5 minutes.
2. Add the stock and the other ingredients except for the chives.
3. Bring to a simmer, then cook over medium heat for 25 minutes, stirring from time to time.

4. Blend the soup using an immersion blender, ladle it into bowls, sprinkle the chives on top, and serve.

Nutrition:

- Calories: 150
- Fat: 3 g
- Carbs: 2 g
- Protein: 6 g

Eggplant Parmesan

Preparation Time:

5 minutes

Cooking Time:

45 minutes

Servings: 8

Ingredients:

- Cooking spray
- 28 ounces crushed tomatoes
- 2 eggplants, sliced into rounds
- 1/4 cups red wine
- ½ Salt and pepper
- 1 teaspoon dried basil
- 2 tablespoons olive oil
- 1 teaspoon dried oregano
- 1 cup onion, chopped
- 1/2 cups parmesan cheese
- 2 cloves garlic, crushed and
- 1 cup mozzarella cheese
- 2 Basil leaves, chopped

Directions:

1. Preheat your oven to 400°F.
2. Merge the ingredients except for the cheese and basil.
3. Spray your baking pan with oil. Simmer for 10 minutes.
4. Arrange the eggplant in the baking pan. Spread the sauce on a baking dish. Season with salt and pepper.
5. Top with the eggplant slices. Roast for 20 minutes.
6. Sprinkle the mozzarella and parmesan on top.
7. Over medium heat, set a pan in place. Attach the oil and cook the onion for 4 minutes.
8. Bake in the oven for 25 minutes.
9. Add in garlic and cook for 2 more minutes.

Nutrition:

- Calories: 192
- Fat: 9 g
- Carbs: 16 g
- Protein: 10 g

Peppers and Lentils Salad

Preparation Time:

10 minutes

Cooking Time:

0 minutes

Servings: 4

Ingredients:

- 14 ounces canned lentils, drained and rinsed
- 2 spring onions, chopped
- 1 red bell pepper, chopped
- 1 green bell pepper, chopped
- 1 tablespoon fresh lime juice
- 1/3 cup coriander, chopped
- 2 teaspoon balsamic vinegar

Directions:

1. In a salad bowl, combine the lentils with the onions, bell peppers, and the rest of the ingredients, toss and serve.

Nutrition:

- Calories: 200
- Fat: 2.45 g
- Fiber: 6.7 g
- Carbs: 10.5 g
- Protein: 5.6 g
- Protein: 10 g

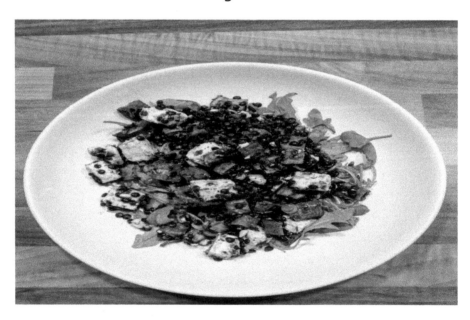

Corn and Tomato Salad

Preparation Time:

10 minutes

Cooking Time:

0 minutes

Servings: 4

Ingredients:

- 2 avocados, pitted, peeled, and cubed
- 1 pint mixed cherry tomatoes, halved
- 2 tablespoons avocado oil
- 1 tablespoon lime juice
- 1/2 teaspoon lime zest, grated
- A pinch of salt and black pepper
- 1/4 cup dill, chopped

Directions:

1. In a salad bowl, mix the avocados with the tomatoes and the rest of the ingredients, toss, and serve cold.

Nutrition:

- Calories: 188
- Fat: 7.3 g
- Fiber: 4.9 g
- Carbs: 6.4 g
- Protein: 6.5 g

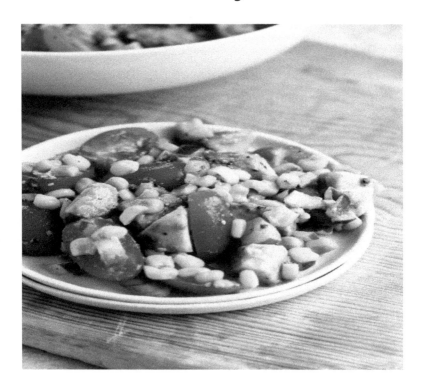

Orange and Cucumber Salad

Preparation Time:

10 minutes

Cooking Time:

0 minutes

Servings: 4

Ingredients:

- 2 cucumbers, sliced
- 1 orange, peeled and cut into segments
- 1 cup cherry tomatoes, halved
- 1 small red onion, chopped
- 3 tablespoons olive oil
- 4 1/2 teaspoons balsamic vinegar
- Salt and black pepper to the taste
- 1 tablespoon lemon juice

Directions:

1. Merge the cucumbers with the orange and the rest of the ingredients, toss and serve cold.

Nutrition:

- Calories: 102
- Fat: 7.5 g
- Fiber: 3 g
- Carbs: 6.1 g
- Protein: 3.4 g

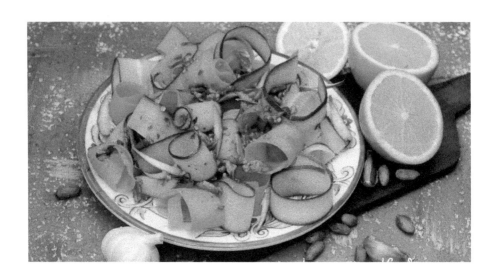

Greek Potato and Corn Salad

Preparation Time:

10 minutes

Cooking Time:

20 minutes

Servings: 2

Ingredients:

- 2 medium potatoes, peeled and cubed
- 2 shallots, chopped
- 1 tablespoon olive oil
- 2 cups corn
- 1 tablespoon dill, chopped
- 1 tablespoon balsamic vinegar
- Salt and black pepper to the taste

Directions:

1. Transfer the potatoes to a pot, add water to cover, bring to a simmer over medium heat, cook for 20 minutes, drain, and transfer to a bowl.
2. Add the shallots and the other ingredients, toss, and serve cold.

Nutrition:

- Calories: 198
- Fat: 5.3 g
- Fiber: 6.5 g
- Carbs: 11.6 g
- Protein: 4.5 g

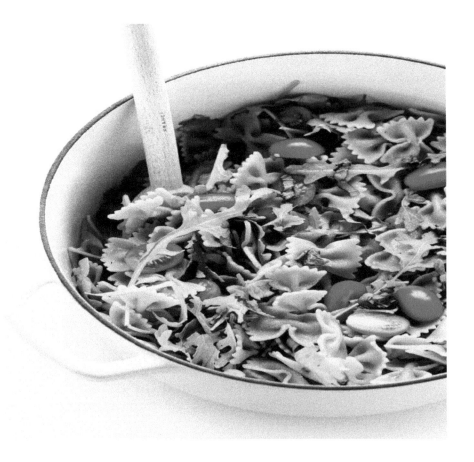

Mint Cabbage Salad

Preparation Time:

10 minutes

Cooking Time:

0 minutes

Servings: 4

Ingredients:

- 1 small red onion, chopped
- 1 tablespoon olive oil
- 2 tablespoons lemon juice
- 1 tablespoon lemon zest, grated
- Salt and black pepper to the taste
- 1 green cabbage head, shredded
- 1/2 cup mint, chopped
- 1/4 cup pistachios, chopped

Directions:

1. Merge the cabbage with the mint, pistachios, and the rest of the ingredients, toss and serve cold.

Nutrition:

- Calories: 101
- Fat: 4.1 g
- Fiber: 3.1 g
- Carbs: 4.5 g
- Protein: 4.6 g

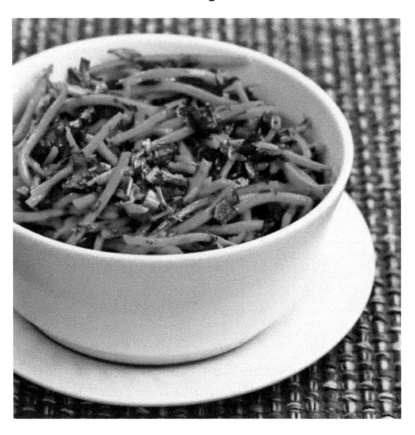

Minty Cauliflower Mix

Preparation Time:

10 minutes

Cooking Time:

0 minutes

Servings: 2

Ingredients:

- 1/2 cups walnuts, chopped
- 2 cups cauliflower florets, steamed
- 1 teaspoon ginger, grated
- 1 garlic clove, minced
- 1 tablespoon mint, chopped
- Juice of 1/2 lemon
- Salt and pepper

Directions:

1. Merge the cauliflower with the walnuts and the rest of the ingredients, toss and serve.

Nutrition:

- Calories: 199
- Fat: 5.6 g
- Fiber: 4.5 g
- Carbs: 8.4 g
- Protein: 3.5 g

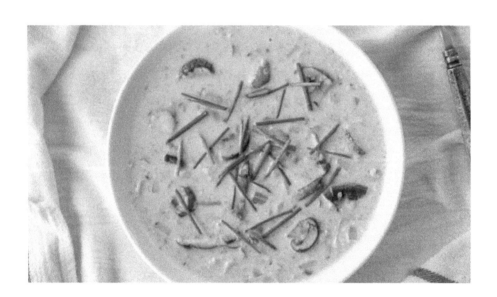

Leeks Salad

Preparation Time:

10 minutes

Cooking Time:

0 minutes

Servings: 4

Ingredients:

- 1 tablespoon olive oil
- 4 leeks, sliced
- 3 garlic cloves, grated
- Salt and white pepper
- 1/2 teaspoon apple cider vinegar
- A drizzle of olive oil
- 1 tablespoon dill, chopped

Directions:

1. In a salad bowl, combine the leeks with the garlic and the rest of the ingredients, toss, and serve cold.

Nutrition:

- Calories: 71
- Fat: 2.1 g
- Fiber: 1.1 g

- Carbs: 1.3 g
- Protein: 2.4 g

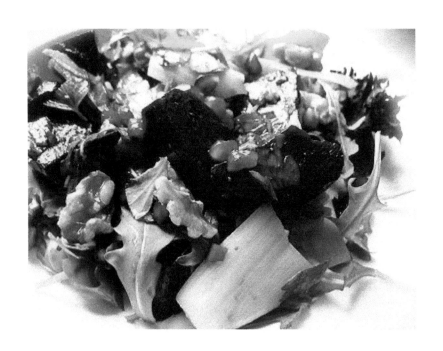

Snow Peas Salad

Preparation Time:

6 hours

Cooking Time:

10 minutes

Servings: 4

Ingredients:

- 3 cups snow peas, trimmed
- 1 1/4 cup bean sprouts
- 1 tablespoon basil, chopped
- 1 tablespoon lime juice
- 1 teaspoon ginger, grated
- 2 spring onions, chopped
- 2 garlic cloves, minced

Directions:

1. Put the snow peas in a pot, add water to cover, bring to a simmer, and cook over medium heat for 10 minutes.
2. Drain the peas, transfer them to a bowl, add the sprouts, and the rest of the ingredients, toss and keep in the fridge for 6 hours before serving.

Nutrition:

- Calories: 200
- Fat: 8.6 g
- Fiber: 3 g
- Carbs: 5.4 g
- Protein: 3.4 g

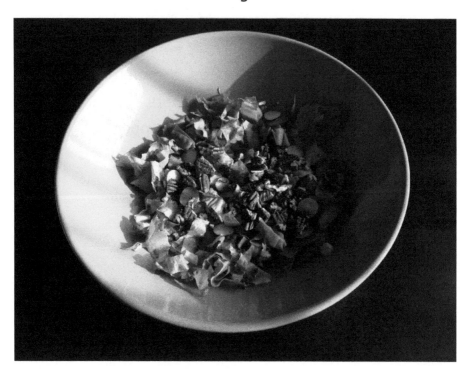

Fennel and Zucchini Mix

Preparation Time:

10 minutes

Cooking Time:

15 minutes

Servings: 4

Ingredients:

- 1 cup fennel bulb, chopped
- 1 sweet onion, chopped
- 1 tablespoon olive oil
- 3 garlic cloves, minced
- 5 cups zucchini, roughly cubed
- 1 cup veggie stock
- Salt and black pepper the taste
- 2 teaspoons white wine vinegar
- 1 teaspoon lemon juice

Directions:

1. Heat the oil and add the onion and the garlic, toss, and sauté for 5 minutes.
2. Merge the rest of the ingredients, toss, cook for 10 minutes more, divide into bowls, and serve.

Nutrition:

- Calories: 193
- Fat: 3 g
- Fiber: 2.4 g
- Carbs: 3 g
- Protein: 2.3 g

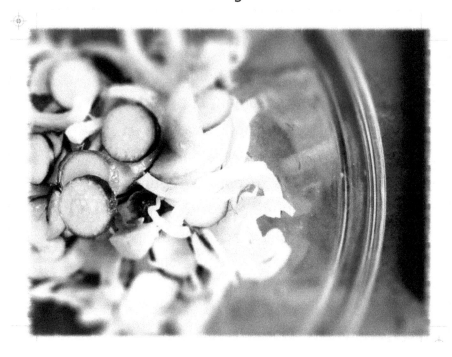

Orange Potato Salad

Preparation Time:

10 minutes

Cooking Time:

40 minutes

Servings: 4

Ingredients:

- 4 sweet potatoes
- 3 tablespoons olive oil
- 1/3 cup orange juice
- 1/2 teaspoon sumac, ground
- 1 tablespoon red wine vinegar
- Salt and black pepper to the taste
- 1 tablespoon orange zest, grated
- 2 tablespoons mint, chopped
- 1/3 cup walnuts, chopped
- 1/3 cup pomegranate seeds

Directions:

1. Put the potatoes on a lined baking sheet, introduce them in the oven at 350°F bake for 40 minutes, cool them down, peel, cut into wedges, and transfer to a bowl.
2. Merge the rest of the ingredients, toss, and serve cold.

Nutrition:

- Calories: 138
- Fat: 3.5 g
- Fiber: 6.2 g
- Carbs: 10.4 g
- Protein: 6.5 g

Avocado Sticks

Preparation Time:

5 minutes

Cooking Time:

10 minutes

Servings: 2

Ingredients:

- 2 avocados
- 1 c. coconut flour
- 2 tsps. black pepper
- 3 egg yolks
- 1½ tbsps. water
- ¼ tsp. salt
- 1 c. vegan butter
- 2 tsps. minced garlic
- ¼ c. chopped parsley
- 1 tbsp. lemon juice

Directions:

1. Place butter in a mixing bowl then adds minced garlic, chopped parsley, and lemon juice to the bowl.
2. Using an electric mixer mix until smooth and fluffy.

3. Transfer the garlic butter to a container with a lid then store in the fridge.

4. Peel the avocados then cut into wedges. Set aside.

5. Put the egg yolks in a mixing bowl then pour water into it.

6. Season with salt and black pepper, then stir until incorporated.

7. Take an avocado wedge then roll in the coconut flour.

8. Dip in the egg mixture then returns back to the coconut flour. Roll until the avocado wedge is completely coated. Repeat with the remaining avocado wedges.

9. Preheat an Air Fryer to 400°F (204°C).

10. Arrange the coated avocado wedges in the Air Fryer basket then cook for 8 minutes or until golden.

11. Remove from the Air Fryer then arrange on a serving dish.

12. Serve with garlic butter then enjoy right away.

Nutrition:

- Calories: 340,
- Fat: 33.8g,
- Protein: 4.5g,
- Carbs: 8.5g

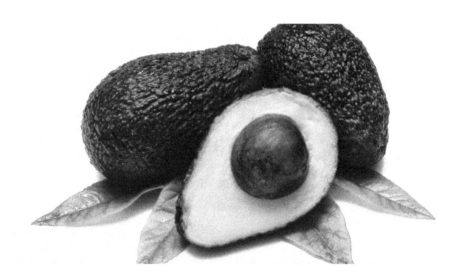

Sizzling Vegetarian Fajitas

Preparation Time:

5 minutes

Cooking Time:

120 minutes

Servings: 2

Ingredients:

- 4 oz. diced green chilies
- ½ tsp. garlic powder
- 3 diced tomatoes
- ¼ tsp. salt
- 1 cored yellow bell pepper,
- 2 tsps. red chili powder
- sliced
- 2 tsps. ground cumin
- 1 cored red bell pepper,
- ½ tsp. dried oregano
- sliced
- 1 ½ tbsps. olive oil
- 1 white onion, peeled and
- sliced

Directions:

1. Take a 6-quarts slow cooker, grease it
2. Plug in the slow cooker; adjust the with a non-stick cooking spray, and
3. Cooking time to 2 hours and let it
4. Add all the ingredients.
5. Cook on the high heat setting or until cooks thoroughly.
6. Stir until it mixes properly and cover STEP 4
7. Serve with tortilla.

Nutrition:

- Calories: 220
- Carbs: 73g,
- Protein: 12g,
- Fats: 8g

Spinach and Feta Pita Bake

Preparation Time:

5 minutes

Cooking Time:

12 minutes

Servings: 3

Ingredients:

- 6 oz. tomato pesto
- 6 whole wheat pita breads
- 2 chopped tomatoes
- ½ c. Kalamata olives
- mushrooms, feta cheese.
- 1 bunch chopped spinach
- 4 sliced mushrooms
- ½ c. crumbled feta cheese
- pepper for seasoning.
- 3 tbsps. olive oil

Directions:

1. Set oven to 350 degrees F.
2. Spread tomato pesto onto one side of each pita bread and place them pesto-side up on a baking sheet.
3. Top pitas with spinach, tomatoes,

4. Sprinkle with olive oil, and add

5. Bake in preheated oven 10-12 minutes or until pitas are crisp.

6. Cut into quarters and serve.

Nutrition:

- 350 Calories,
- Protein, 17g
- Fat: 41g
- Carbs 152

Quinoa And Spinach Cakes

Preparation Time:

5 minutes

Cooking Time:

9 minutes

Servings: 2

Ingredients:

- 2 c. cooked quinoa
- 1 c. chopped baby spinach
- 1 egg
- 2 tbsps. minced parsley
- 1 tsp. minced garlic
- 1 carrot, peeled and shredded
- 1 chopped onion
- ¼ c. oat milk
- ¼ c. parmesan cheese, grated
- 1 c. breadcrumbs
- sea salt
- ground black peppers

Directions:

1. In a mixing bowl, mix all ingredients.
2. Season with salt and pepper to taste.
3. Preheat your Air Fryer to 390°F.

4. Scoop ¼ cup of quinoa and spinach mixture and place in the Air Fryer cooking basket.

5. Cook in batches until browned for about 8 minutes.

6. Serve and enjoy!

Nutrition:

- Calories: 188,
- Fat: 4.4 g,
- Carbs: 31.2g,
- Protein: 8.1g

Garlicky Kale & Pea Saute

Preparation Time:

5 minutes

Cooking Time:

8 minutes

Servings: 2

Ingredients:

- 2 sliced garlic cloves
- 1 chopped hot red chile
- 2 tbsps. olive oil
- 2 bunches chopped kale
- 1 lb. frozen peas

Directions:

1. In a saucepot, mix the ingredients except peas. Cook until the kale becomes tender for about 6 minutes.
2. Add peas and cook for 2 more minutes.

Nutrition:

- Calories 85,
- Fats 11g
- Protein 158

Mashed Cauliflower

Preparation Time:

5 minutes

Cooking Time:

6 minutes

Servings: 4

Ingredients:

- 1 head cauliflower head
- 3 tbsps. melt vegetarian butter
- 1 c. water
- ¼ c. pepper
- ½ tsp. salt

Directions:

1. Chop the cauliflower and place inside the steamer basket.
2. Pour the water into the Pressure Pot and lower the basket.
3. Close the lid, set it to MANUAL, and cook at high pressure for 4 minutes.
4. Do a quick pressure release.
5. Mash the cauliflower with a potato masher or in a food processor and stir in the remaining ingredients.
6. Serve and enjoy!

Nutrition:

- Calories: 113;
- Fat: 5.9 g;
- Carbs: 4.1 g;
- Protein: 3 g 161

Sun-dried Tomato Pesto

Preparation Time:

5 minutes

Cooking Time:

11 minutes

Servings: 5

Ingredients:

- 1 c. fresh basil leaves
- 6 oz. sun-dried tomatoes
- 1 tbsp. lemon juice
- ½ tsp. salt
- ¼ c. olive oil
- ¼ c. almonds
- 3 minced garlic cloves
- ½ tsp. chopped red pepper
- 8 oz. pasta

Directions:

1. Cook the pasta according to the given instructions.
2. For making, the pesto, toasts the almonds over medium flame in a small skillet for around 4 minutes.

3. In a blender, put sun-dried tomatoes, basil, garlic, lemon juice, salt, red pepper flakes, and toasted almonds and blend it.

4. While blending adds olive oil in it and blend it until it converts in the form of a pesto. flakes

5. Now coat the pasta with the pesto and serve it.

Nutrition:

- Calories 256,
- Fat 13.7g,
- Carbs 28.1g,
- Protein 6.7g 162

Grilled Zucchini

Preparation Time:

5 minutes

Cooking Time:

10 minutes

Servings: 2

Ingredients:

- 4 zucchinis, sliced
- 1 tbsp. olive oil
- salt and pepper
- 1 c. tomatoes, chopped
- 1 tbsp. mint, chopped
- 1 tsp. red wine vinegar

Directions:

1. Preheat your grill.
2. Coat the zucchini with oil and season with salt and pepper.
3. Grill for 4 minutes per side.
4. Mix the remaining ingredients in a bowl.
5. Top the grilled zucchini with the minty salsa.

Nutrition:

- Calories 71,
- Fat 5 g,
- Carbs 6 g,
- Protein 2 g 170

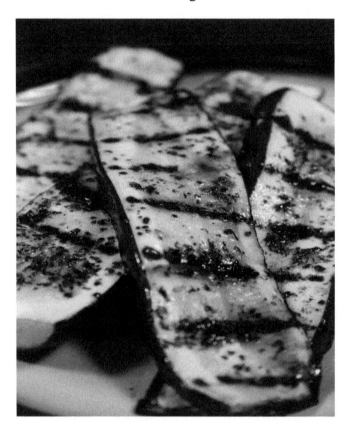

Eggplant Italiano

Preparation Time:

5 minutes

Cooking Time:

5 minutes

Servings: 8

Ingredients:

- 2½ lbs. eggplant, cubed
- 4 celery stalks, cut into 1-inch
- 2 sliced onions
- 7½ oz. canned tomato sauce
- 2 cans (16 ounce each) diced
- 2 tbsps. olive oil, divided
- 1 c. olives pitted and halved
- 4 tbsps. balsamic vinegar
- 2 tbsps. drained capers
- 1 tbsp. maple syrup
- 2 tsps. dried basil
- salt
- pepper
- basil leaves to garnish

Directions:

1. Add all the ingredients into the
2. Pressure Pot. Stir to mix well
3. Close the lid. Select MANUAL and cook at high pressure for 4 minutes.
4. When the cooking is complete, do a quick pressure release.
5. Garnish with fresh basil and serve over rice or noodles.

Nutrition:

- Calories: 127;
- Fat: 5.8 g;
-
- Carbs: 11.6; Protein: 3 g 174

Balsamic-Glazed Roasted

Preparation Time:

5 minutes

Cooking Time:

75 minutes

Servings: 4

Ingredients:

- 1 head cauliflower
- ½ lb. green beans, trimmed
- 1 peeled red onion, wedged
- 2 c. cherry tomatoes
- ½ tsp. salt
- ¼ c. brown sugar
- 3 tbsps. olive oil
- 1 c. balsamic vinegar
- 2 tbsps. chopped parsley, for

Directions:

1. Place cauliflower florets in a baking dish, add tomatoes, green beans, and onion wedges around it, season with salt, and drizzle with oil.

2. Pour vinegar in a saucepan, stir in sugar, bring the mixture to a boil and simmer for 15 minutes until reduced by half.

3. Brush the sauce generously over cauliflower florets and then roast for 1 hour at 400 degrees f until cooked, brushing sauce frequently.

4. When done, garnish vegetables with parsley and then serve.

Nutrition:

- Calories: 86,
- Fat: 5.7 g,
- Carbs: 7.7 g,
- Protein: 3.1 g 177

Charred Green Beans with Mustard

Preparation Time:

5 minutes

Cooking Time:

20 minutes

Servings: 2

Ingredients:

- 1 teaspoon whole-grain mustard
- 1/8 teaspoon salt
- 1/8 teaspoon black pepper
- 1½ tablespoons olive oil, divided
- ½ pound green beans, trimmed
- ½ tablespoon red-wine vinegar
- 1/8 cup toasted hazelnuts, chopped

Directions:

1. Preheat a grill on high heat and grease a grill pan.
2. Mix green beans with ½ tablespoon of olive oil in a pan.
3. Transfer to the grill pan and grill the beans for about 8 minutes.
4. Mix the beans with mustard, olive oil, vinegar, salt and black pepper.
5. Top with hazelnuts and serve hot.

Nutrition:

- Calories 181
- Total Fat 14.6 g
- Saturated Fat 2.3 g
- Cholesterol 97 mg
- Total Carbs 8.5 g
- Dietary Fiber 6.1 g
- Sugar 2.4 g
- Protein 2.8 g

Lemony Mushroom and Herb Rice

Preparation Time:

5 minutes

Cooking Time:

20 minutes

Servings: 8

Ingredients:

- 4 large garlic cloves, finely chopped
- ¼ cup parsley, chopped
- 6 tablespoons chives, snipped
- 2½ cups chestnut mushrooms, diced
- 2 cups long grain rice
- 4 tablespoons olive oil
- 2 lemons, zested

Direction:

1. Boil water with salt in a pan and add rice.
2. Cook for about 10 minutes while stirring continuously and drain them through a sieve.
3. Sauté mushrooms for about 5 minutes and stir in the garlic cloves.

4. Sauté for about 1 minute and toss in chives, parsley, lemon zest and drained rice.

5. Dish out to serve and enjoy.

Nutrition:

- Calories 281
- Total Fat 8.9 g
- Saturated Fat 1.4 g
- Cholesterol 0 mg
- Total Carbs 43.6 g
- Dietary Fiber 5.4 g
- Sugar 0.8 g
- Protein 9 g

Smoky Roasted Vegetables

Preparation Time:

10 minutes

Cooking Time:

1 hour 40 minutes

Servings: 4

Ingredients:

- ½ orange bell pepper, sliced
- 1 bay leaf
- 1 small red onion, sliced into rounds and separated
- ½ summer squash, cut into 3-inch sticks
- ½ teaspoon sea salt, divided
- 1/6 cup extra-virgin olive oil
- 2 small tomatoes, sliced
- ½ yellow bell pepper, sliced
- ½ zucchini, cut into 3-inch sticks
- 1 sprig fresh thyme
- ½ tablespoon balsamic vinegar
- ½ tablespoon red-wine vinegar
- ½ eggplant, cut into 3-inch sticks
- 2 sprigs fresh parsley
- 2 garlic cloves, divided

Direction:

1. Preheat the oven to 360 degrees F and lightly grease a baking dish.
2. Season all the vegetables with salt and transfer to the baking dish.
3. Tie parsley, thyme and bay leaf with a kitchen string and place them at the center of the seasoned vegetables.
4. Drizzle with oil and top with garlic cloves.
5. Transfer in the oven and bake for about 1 hour 15 minutes.
6. Drizzle with vinegar and serve immediately.

Nutrition:

- Calories 231
- Total Fat 17.5 g
- Saturated Fat 2.5 g
- Cholesterol 0 mg
- Total Carbs 19.6 g
- Dietary Fiber 7.3 g
- Sugar 10.6 g
- Protein 3.6 g

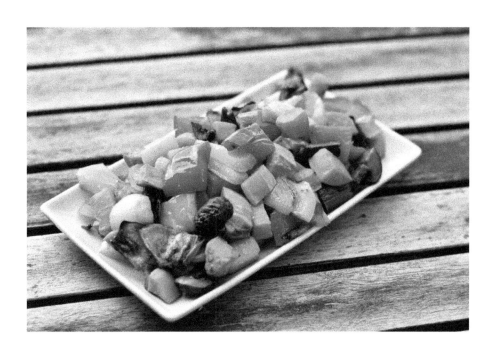

Lightning Source UK Ltd.
Milton Keynes UK
UKHW020634140621
385477UK00005B/130